Monkeypox : Fact or Fiction

Kimberly A. Ashby

Table of contents

Introduction

While clinically less severe than smallpox, monkeypox is a viral zoonosis (a virus that spreads from animals to people). It has symptoms that are comparable to those of smallpox. Monkeypox has replaced smallpox as the most significant orthopoxvirus for public health since smallpox was eradicated in 1980 and smallpox vaccinations were subsequently discontinued. Primarily affecting central and west Africa, monkeypox has been spreading into cities and is often seen close to tropical rainforests. Numerous rodent species and non-human primates serve as hosts for animals.

An infectious viral illness called monkeypox may affect both humans and certain other animals. Fever, enlarged lymph nodes, and a rash that develops blisters before crusting over are all symptoms. Five to twenty-one days pass from exposure to the start of symptoms. Symptoms last between two and four weeks on average. Mild signs might be present, or it could happen with no documented symptoms. It has been discovered that not all outbreaks exhibit the typical presentation of fever and muscular aches followed by enlarged glands and lesions all developing at the same time. Particularly in youngsters, expectant women, or those with weakened immune systems, cases may be severe.

The virus that causes the illness is called the monkeypox virus, and it belongs to the genus Orthopoxvirus. This genus also contains the smallpox virus and the variola virus. The sickness caused by clade II, previously known as the West African clade, in humans is less severe than the disease caused by the Central African (Congo basin) type.

By handling diseased meat or via bites or scratches, it may be transmitted from infected animals. Human-to-human transmission may take place by contact with contaminated items or bodily fluids, through tiny droplets, or perhaps through the airborne route. People may transfer the virus from the moment symptoms appear until all lesions have crusted over and fallen off, and there may still be signs of dissemination for up to a week after that. Testing a lesion for the virus' DNA will confirm the diagnosis.

No recognized treatment exists. According to 1988 research, smallpox vaccination was around 85% effective at reducing the severity of the illness and avoiding infection in close contact. With limited availability, a more recent smallpox and monkeypox vaccination based on modified vaccinia Ankara has been authorized.

Regular hand washing and avoiding ill people and animals are further precautions. During epidemics, antiviral medications like cidofovir and tecovirimat, vaccinia immune globulin, and the smallpox vaccination may be utilized. The majority of infected people recover within a few weeks without therapy since the sickness is often mild. The risk of mortality is estimated to range from 1% to 10%, however, since 2017, there haven't been many fatalities linked to monkeypox.

It is believed that several animal species serve as the virus's natural reservoir.

The frequency and intensity of outbreaks have considerably risen since the 1980s, even though it was originally believed to be rare in humans. This could be due to diminishing immunity as a consequence of the cessation of regular smallpox vaccinations.

The first human cases were discovered in the Democratic Republic of the Congo in 1970. (DRC).

It is endemic in the DRC, with isolated instances throughout Central and West Africa. The 2022 monkeypox epidemic, which was originally discovered in the United Kingdom in May 2022 and later confirmed in at least 74 nations on all continents except Antarctica, is the first instance of extensive community transmission outside of Africa. With more than 16,000 cases documented in 75 countries and territories, the World Health Organization (WHO) designated the epidemic a Public Health Emergency of International Concern (PHEIC) on July 23, 2022.

Chapter 1: History Of Monkeypox

In Copenhagen, Denmark, laboratory monkeys were the first to get monkeypox, which was thereafter recognized as a unique e disease. The first known human cases were six unvaccinated toddlers in 1970 who were part of the smallpox eradication campaign. The first case was a 9-month-old kid in the Democratic Republic of the Congo (formerly Zaire). The rest, including three playmates, were in Sierra Leone and Liberia. It was noticed that it spreads less quickly than smallpox.

In the DRC, nearly 300 cases of human monkeypox were documented between 1981 and 1986, with animal interaction accounting for the bulk of these cases. 88% of cases of the illness that returned to the DRC in 1996 were spread from person to person. In tropical Central and West Africa, small viral epidemics with fatality rates around 10% and rates of secondary human-to-human transmission around the same proportion are common. Up until 2003, when monkeypox broke out in the US, the illness was exclusive to the rain forests of Western and Central Africa humans. All instances were linked to imported ill rats from Ghana. The disease was contracted by local prairie dogs, who then infected their owners. There were no fatalities and the illness was deemed to be mild. The illness was documented in 10 African nations between 1970 and 2019; predominantly in Central and West Africa.

In 2018, two unrelated Nigerian travelers were found to have monkeypox in the UK.

In the UK during that year, the first human-to-human transmission outside of Africa was verified.

This individual was a healthcare professional who could have become sick by using contaminated sheets. Additionally, cases involving visitors to Singapore and Israel were mentioned. More incidents occurred in the UK in 2019 and 2021.

In June 2022, the World Health Organization said that, in keeping with its goal to prevent false links with particular locations or animals, it will come up with a new name for the illness. The first monkeypox fatality in India was reported on July 31, 2022. The victim was a 22-year-old guy who had just returned from the United Arab Emirates.

Monkeypox Outbreak

In the Democratic Republic of the Congo, where smallpox had been eradicated in 1968, a 9-month-old child was the first person to be diagnosed with human monkeypox. Since then, human cases have progressively been recorded from central and west Africa, with the majority of cases coming from the rural, rainforest parts of the Congo Basin, mainly in the Democratic Republic of the Congo.

Benin, Cameroon, the Central African Republic, the Democratic Republic of the Congo, Gabon, Cote d'Ivoire, Liberia, Nigeria, the Republic of the Congo, Sierra Leone, and South Sudan are the 11 African nations where human cases of monkeypox have been documented since 1970. The unknown is the real cost of monkeypox. For instance, an epidemic with a lower case fatality ratio and a higher attack rate than typical was recorded in the Democratic Republic of the Congo from 1996–1997.

Monkeypox and chickenpox outbreaks that occurred simultaneously in this instance might be explained by actual or perceived modifications in the dynamics of transmission produced by the varicella virus, which is not an orthopoxvirus. Over 500 suspected cases, over 200 confirmed cases, and a case fatality rate of about 3% have been reported in Nigeria since 2017. Cases are still being reported today.

Given that it affects the rest of the globe in addition to nations in west and central Africa, monkeypox is a disease of worldwide public health significance. The first monkeypox epidemic outside of Africa occurred in the United States of America in 2003, and contact with pet prairie dogs that had the disease was to blame. These pets had been kept alongside dormice and pouched rats from Ghana that were brought from the Gambia. Over 70 cases of monkeypox were brought on by this epidemic in the US. Travelers from Nigeria to Israel in September 2018, the UK in September 2018, December 2019, May 2021, and May 2022, Singapore in May 2019, and the United States of America in July and November 2021 have also been reported to have monkeypox.

Monkeypox cases were found in several non-endemic nations in May 2022. Studies are being conducted right now to learn more about the epidemiology, sources of illness, and patterns of transmission.

Chapter 2: Signs, Symptoms and Epidemiology of Monkeypox

A person can be infected with monkeypox without showing any symptoms. Monkeypox symptoms tend to begin 5 to 21 days after infection, with early symptoms including headache, muscle pains, fever, and fatigue, initially resembling influenza. Within a few days of the fever, lesions characteristically appear on the face before appearing on the trunk and then elsewhere such as palms of the hands and soles of the feet.

The disease can resemble chickenpox, measles, and smallpox but is distinguished by the presence of swollen glands which may appear behind the ear, below the jaw, in the neck, or the groin, before the onset of the rash. Many cases in the 2022 monkeypox outbreak presented with genital and peri-anal lesions, fever, swollen lymph nodes, and pain when swallowing, with some patients manifesting only single sores from the disease.

Three-quarters of affected people have lesions on the palms and soles, more than two-thirds in the mouth, a third on the genitals, and one in five have lesions in the eyes. They begin as small flat spots, before becoming small bumps which then fill with at first clear fluid and then yellow fluid, which subsequently burst and scab over, persisting for around ten days. There may be a few lesions or several thousand, sometimes merging to produce large lesions. After healing, the lesions may leave pale marks before becoming dark scars.

An unwell person may remain so for two to four weeks.

Epidemiology

In the settlement of Basankusu, Équateur Province, the Democratic Republic of the Congo (formerly Zaire), monkeypox was first connected to the condition as a disease in people in 1970. Although it was long believed to be rare in humans, instances have risen since the 1980s, probably due to diminishing immunity after the end of regular smallpox vaccination.

In the DRC/Zaire, WHO monitoring between 1981 and 1986 tallied 338 confirmed cases and 33 fatalities (CFR 9.8%). A second human disease epidemic was discovered in DRC/Zaire in 1996–1997, and between 1991 and 1999, 511 cases were documented there. The disease's Clade I genetic subgroup, which is still prevalent in the DRC, has a higher CFR than the other subgroup in Western Africa.

The case fatality rate (CFR) for prior epidemics was between 3% and 6% by May 2022, whereas it was less than 1% for the outbreak in 2022. Before the monkeypox epidemic in Europe in 2022, no human-to-human transmission has been identified. The first monkeypox epidemic outside of Africa occurred in 2003 among prairie dog owners in the Midwest of the United States. This outbreak was caused by Clade II. According to reports, 71 persons contracted the disease, however, none of them died.

Monkeypox has historically only existed in the environment of tropical rainforests as of 2018. The trend was halted in 2005, however, when 49 instances in Sudan (regions that are now South Sudan) were documented with no deaths. According to the genetic study, the virus was imported, most likely from the DRC, and did not originate in Sudan.

In Central and West Africa, namely the Democratic Republic of the Congo, many more instances of monkeypox have been documented: 2000 cases per year are recorded between 2011 and 2014. Realistic projections of the number of monkeypox cases over time are hampered by the sometimes fragmentary and unsubstantiated nature of the data that has been gathered. However, it was claimed that as of 2018, both the recorded cases and the geographic distribution of monkeypox have expanded.

U.S. epidemic in 2003

In May 2003, a small kid who had been bitten by a prairie dog bought at a neighborhood swap meet close to Milwaukee, Wisconsin, had a fever and rash. Through June 20, 2003, a total of 71 cases of monkeypox were documented. A Texas exotic animal distributor's shipment of Gambian pouched rats from Accra, Ghana in April 2003 was the source of all cases. No one perished. The diagnosis of human monkeypox was supported by serological research and electron microscopy.

Typical prodromal signs of monkeypox were fever, headaches, muscular pains, chills, and drenching sweats. A third or so of those who were afflicted coughed ineffectively. A papular rash that commonly proceeded through phases of vesiculation, pustulation, umbilication, and crusting appeared 1–10 days after this prodromal phase. Early lesions had developed into ulcers in some patients.

On the head, trunk, and limbs, there were rashes and sores. On the palms, soles, and extremities of several of the patients were primary and secondary lesions. Some people's rashes seemed to be widespread. People often developed rash lesions at various stages after the rash started. Everyone who was impacted claimed to have had direct or intimate contact with prairie dogs that were subsequently shown to have the monkeypox virus.

The Nigerian epidemic, 2017–2019

Only 10 human monkeypox infections were documented in Nigeria between 1971 and 1978, according to the Nigeria Centre for Disease Control (NCDC).

39 years after its last documented case, human monkeypox reemerged in Nigeria in September 2017. With 118 confirmed cases, the ensuing human monkeypox epidemic in Nigeria in 2017–18 was, at the time, the virus's largest-ever clade II outbreak. In contrast to other outbreaks

of this lineage, infection was mostly among young male adults, and it seems that human-to-human transmission happened easily. An infant and four HIV/AIDS patients were among the seven recorded fatalities (case fatality rate: 6%; five male, two female). In addition, a second-trimester pregnant lady with monkeypox miscarried on her own.

According to the Niger Delta University Teaching Hospital, many of its young adult patients also had genital ulcers, syphilis, and HIV infection. South and southeast Nigeria were affected by the monkeypox outbreak, which certain states and the federal government of Nigeria were attempting to suppress. By the end of 2017, it has expanded to the following states: Akwa Ibom, Abia, Bayelsa, Benue, Cross River, Delta, Edo, Ekiti, Enugu, Imo, Lagos, Nasarawa, Oyo, Plateau, Rivers, and Federal Capital Territory.

As of May 2019, the epidemic was continuing strong throughout many states after beginning in September 2017.

After returning from Lagos and Ibadan, instances of monkeypox were recorded by the Centers for Disease Control and Prevention.

According to Agam Rao, a medical officer in the CDC's Division of Pathogens and High Consequence Pathology, all cases documented outside of Africa since 2018 have originated in Nigeria.

Oyewale Tomori noted in a 2021 article that the number of monkeypox infections in Nigeria until 2021 was probably under-reported since a sizable portion of the populace had been avoiding healthcare facilities out of concern about catching COVID-19.

558 instances were verified throughout 32 states and the Federal Capital Territory between 2017 and 2022, according to a report published by the Nigerian government in May 2022. Monkeypox was most prevalent in Rivers State, then Bayelsa and Lagos. With 8 recorded fatalities, the case fatality ratio was 3.5%. A National Technical

Working Group was established by NCDC in 2022 to improve infection reporting and monitoring.

United Kingdom cases from 2018 and 2019.
The first case of monkeypox in the United Kingdom was discovered in September 2018. The individual, a citizen of Nigeria, is thought to have acquired monkeypox in Nigeria before traveling to the United Kingdom. The individual was staying at a military installation in Cornwall when they were transferred to the Royal Free Hospital's specialized infectious illness unit, according to Public Health England. The individual contacted others who had come into touch with him after contracting the illness.

In the town of Blackpool, a second case was verified, and a third case involved a Blackpool-based medical professional who treated the second victim. On December 3, 2019, a person in southwest England was diagnosed with monkeypox, marking the fourth incidence of the year. They were making their way from Nigeria to the UK.

Singapore case in 2019

On May 8, 2019, a 38-year-old man from Nigeria was admitted to the National Centre for Infectious Diseases in Singapore and placed in an isolation ward after being identified as the nation's first monkeypox case. 22 persons were placed under quarantine as a consequence. Possible connections between the case and a concurrent epidemic in Nigeria exist.

2021 instances in the US and the UK

Public Health Wales in the UK discovered three cases of monkeypox on May 24 in a single home. In a speech to MPs, Health Secretary Matt Hancock also disclosed the incidents. After arriving from Nigeria, the index case had a diagnosis on May 24. On June 2, the second case was reported, and on June 24, the third. Tecovirimat was administered to a female adult patient who was one of the three patients. She was released from the hospital on day 7 of tecovirimat and continued her second week of therapy at home.

An American who had just returned from a vacation to Nigeria was given the diagnosis of monkeypox on July 14 in the US. The virus was determined by further testing to belong to clade II. When receiving tecovirimat treatment in a hospital setting for 32 days, the patient was released after the monkeypox virus DNA was no longer present in any lingering skin lesions.

2022 epidemic

In May 2022, it was determined that monkeypox, a viral illness, was still on the rise.

The first case was discovered on May 6, 2022, in a person with travel ties to Nigeria, and the first cluster of cases was discovered there (where the disease is endemic). For the first time outside of Central and West Africa, monkeypox was extensively distributed during the pandemic. Cases began to be recorded from an expanding number of nations and areas starting on May 18, mostly in Europe but also in North and South America, Asia, Africa, and Oceania. Tedros Adhanom Ghebreyesus, the head of the World Health Organization (WHO), declared the epidemic a public health emergency of worldwide concern on July 23. (PHEIC). [105] 42,258 confirmed cases of monkeypox were reported worldwide as of August 21. Most of these cases were in places where monkeypox had not previously been reported.

Complications

Complications include secondary infections, pneumonia, sepsis, encephalitis, and loss of vision with a severe eye infection. If infection occurs during pregnancy, stillbirth or birth defects may occur. The disease may be milder in people vaccinated against smallpox in childhood. In other animals

The disease has also been reported in dormice, tree squirrels, rope squirrels, and non-human primates. Rodents such as rats and mice are likely susceptible but not known. Signs and symptoms in animals vary among different species. Monkeypox-infected Gambian pouched rats may have mild symptoms. During the 2003 US outbreak, affected prairie dogs presented with fever, cough, sore eyes, poor feeding, and rash. Non-human primates present similarly.

They may have breathing problems, facial swelling, mouth ulcers, and swollen glands. In cynomolgus monkeys, the time from exposure to symptoms was noted to be around a week. Rabbits and rodents typically present with fever, cough, runny nose, sore eyes, and swollen glands. They develop small bumps that fill with yellow fluid and may have patches of hair loss and pneumonia. Spreading among animals occurs via the fecal-oral route and through the nose, through wounds, and eating infected meat. Death is more likely in baby monkeys. The CDC recommends that animals exposed to monkeypox be quarantined for six weeks.

Human Transmission

By being bitten, scratched, eating bush meat, or coming into touch with an infected animal's body fluids or lesion material, humans may get infected by animals. The respiratory system, mucous membranes of the eyes, nose, and mouth, as well as breaks in the skin are considered to be entry sites for the virus.

When a human becomes sick, infection among other people often occurs, posing a significant risk of infection for family members and medical personnel. The virus may be transmitted from one person to another by respiratory (airborne) contact, direct contact with body fluids from an infected person, or from a pregnant woman to her fetus. Given that the contagious monkeypox virus can be isolated from samples of semen, there are signs that transmission may happen during sexual intercourse.

Long-term monkeypox viral shedding in seminal fluids raises the prospect of a genital reservoir. If the virus may spread via vaginal secretions is unknown.

Even with adequate personal protective equipment, the virus may spread through fomites or by indirect contact with lesion material, such as through contaminated bedding, most commonly through inhalation. Sharing a bed or room or using the same utensils as an infected individual are risk factors for transmission. Factors that involve the passage of the virus to the oral mucosa are linked to an increased likelihood of transmission. It is still unknown whether those who do not have monkeypox symptoms may transmit the virus.

The strain that caused the epidemic in 2022 is still the subject of continuing study into its mode of transmission, however, it is not believed to vary from previous clade II strains.

Animals Transmission

Direct contact with the blood, body fluids and cutaneous or mucosal lesions of infected animals may result in animal-to-human (zoonotic) transfer. Numerous animals in Africa, including rope squirrels, tree squirrels, Gambian pouched rats, dormice, several kinds of monkeys, and others, have shown signs of monkeypox virus infection. Rodents are the most plausible candidates for the monkeypox natural reservoir, however, this has not yet been determined. Eating undercooked meat and other diseased animal products is a potential risk factor. People who live in or close to forests may be indirectly or minimally exposed to diseased animals.

Close contact with respiratory secretions, skin sores on an infected person, or recently contaminated items may cause human-to-human transmission. Health professionals, family members, and other close contacts of current patients are more at risk because droplet respiratory particles often need extended face-to-face contact. The number of person-to-person infections in a community's longest recorded chain of transmission has increased from 6 to 9 in recent years. This could be an indication of a general decline in immunity brought on by the end of smallpox vaccination campaigns.

Congenital monkeypox may result through transmission via the placenta, which can also happen during intimate contact during labor and after delivery. Although close physical contact is a recognized risk factor for transmission, it is not known at this time whether monkeypox may particularly spread via sexual intercourse. Studies are required to comprehend this danger better.

Chapter 3: What causes monkeypox?

When you come into touch with an animal or a person who is infected with the virus, you might develop monkeypox. Animals may transmit diseases to people by biting or scratching people, or by coming into direct touch with their blood, body fluids, or lesions from an affected animal (sores).

Although less frequent, monkeypox may transmit from person to person. When you come into touch with the sores, scabs, respiratory droplets, or oral secretions of an infected individual, often via close, personal interactions like hugging, kissing, or intercourse, person-to-person spread (transmission) takes place. Although a study is underway, it is unclear if the virus is spread by semen or vaginal secretions.

Monkeypox may also spread by contact with recently contaminated items, such as clothes, bedding, and other linens used by an infected human or an infected animal.

The monkeypox virus, a double-stranded DNA virus belonging to the genus Orthopoxvirus and family Poxviridae, is what causes monkeypox in both people and animals. The virus, which is most prevalent in tropical rainforest areas of Central and West Africa, was initially discovered in captive monkeys. The virus has two subtypes, clade I and clade II (formerly Congo Basin and West African clades, matching the geographical areas).

The virus has also been found in African squirrels, dormice (Graphiurus spp.), and Gambian pouched rats (Cricetomys Gambians) in addition to monkeys (Heliosciurus, and Funisciurus). One significant route of transmission to humans may be the consumption of these animals as food.

A kind of double-stranded DNA virus known as the monkeypox virus (MPV, MPXV, or hMPXV) causes monkeypox in both humans and other animals. It is a member of the family Poxviridae and the genus Orthopoxvirus. Together with the variola (VARV), cowpox (CPX), and vaccinia (VACV) viruses, the monkeypox virus is one of the human orthopoxviruses. It is neither a direct ancestor nor a direct descendent of the smallpox-causing variola virus. Smallpox and monkeypox are similar, but monkeypox has a milder rash and a lower fatality rate.

Risk Elements

First off, anybody who has close physical contact with a person exhibiting viral symptoms or a virus-infected animal is at risk of becoming ill. Those who have had a smallpox vaccination are at low risk of developing the illness, but they must use the appropriate precautions to prevent monkeypox.

Newborns, adults with weakened immune systems, and children and adolescents who have not received the smallpox vaccine are at particularly high risk of getting the illness.

Because of their extended viral exposure, health personnel are also susceptible to the infection.

Chapter 4: Diagnosis and Treatment of Monkeypox

Other rash disorders such as chickenpox, measles, bacterial skin infections, scabies, syphilis, and medication-related allergies must be taken into account when making a clinical differential diagnosis. As a clinical characteristic, lymphadenopathy during the prodromal stage of the disease may help differentiate monkeypox from chickenpox or smallpox.

Health professionals should get the right sample and arrange for it to be delivered securely to a lab with the right equipment if monkeypox is detected. The kind of laboratory test used and the kind and quality of the material used to determine whether monkeypox is confirmed. As a result, specimens should be sent and handled in line with local, state, and federal regulations. Given its precision and sensitivity, polymerase chain reaction (PCR) is the primary laboratory test.

The best diagnostic samples for monkeypox come from skin lesions, such as dry crusts and the liquid that comes from vesicles and pustules. A biopsy is a possibility when it is possible. Lesion samples must be maintained cool and stored in a dry, sterile tube without a viral transport medium. Due to the brief period of viremia about the date of specimen collection after symptoms begin, PCR blood tests are often inconclusive and should not be regularly obtained from patients.

Antigen and antibody detection techniques do not offer proof of monkeypox-specific infection because orthopoxviruses are serologically cross-reactive. Therefore, in cases where resources are few, serology and antigen detection procedures are not advised for diagnosis or case inquiry. Furthermore, recent or distant immunization with a vaccinia-based vaccine (for example, anybody immunized before the eradication of smallpox, or more recently owing to heightened risk, such as orthopoxvirus laboratory employees) may result in false positive findings.

The following patient data must be included with the specimens to interpret test results: a) age; b) date of start of fever; c) date of the specimen collection; d) date of the current condition of the patient (stage of rash), and e) date of the beginning of rash.

There are many ways to identify monkeypox:

Medical history: If you have been to a nation where the illness is widespread, the doctor may question you about your medical history.

Lab tests: During this treatment, the doctor may test fluid from lesions or dried scabs. The virus may be examined in these samples using a polymerase chain reaction (PCR) assay.

They could also do a biopsy, which involves the removal of some skin tissue and testing it for the virus.

Treatment

Tecovirimat has received approval for the treatment of many poxviruses, including monkeypox, in the European Union and the United States. If necessary, BMJ Best Practice advises using supportive care in addition to tecovirimat or the smallpox medication brincidofovir as the first line of antiviral therapy (including antipyretic, fluid balance, and oxygenation). If subsequent bacterial or varicella zoster infection is suspected, empirical antibiotic treatment or aciclovir may be utilized.

Prevention

Because smallpox and monkeypox viruses are closely related, and because the vaccination shields animals against deadly monkeypox challenges during experiments, it is expected that the vaccine will protect against human monkeypox infection. Because systematic smallpox vaccination was stopped after smallpox was eradicated, this has not been definitively shown in people.

In Africa, it has been noted that the smallpox vaccination lowers the risk of monkeypox among those who have already received the shot. Monkeypox is more common because exposed people have a decreased level of immunity to poxviruses. It is related to the progressive rise in the number of unvaccinated people as well as to the fading cross-protective immunity among those immunized before 1980 when bulk smallpox vaccines were stopped.

The United States Centers for Disease Control and Prevention (CDC) advises that anybody engaged in caring for sick people or animals or doing research into monkeypox outbreaks be vaccinated against smallpox to protect against monkeypox. People should also be vaccinated if they have come into close or personal contact with people or animals who have been diagnosed with monkeypox.

Pre-exposure immunization is not advised by the CDC for veterinary professionals, veterinary assistants, or animal control officers who have not been exposed unless they are engaged in field research. No vaccination against smallpox or monkeypox has been authorized for use during pregnancy.

Before treating an infected patient, healthcare professionals are advised to put on a complete complement of personal protective equipment (PPE), according to the CDC. This consists of a robe, mask, pair of goggles, and a filtering disposable respirator (such as an N95). To prevent potential contact with others, an infected individual should be segregated, ideally in a negative air pressure chamber or at the very least a private exam room. and Transmission

Direct contact with the blood, body fluids and cutaneous or mucosal lesions of infected animals may result in animal-to-human (zoonotic) transfer. Numerous animals in Africa, including rope squirrels, tree squirrels, Gambian pouched rats, dormice, several kinds of monkeys, and others, have shown signs of monkeypox virus infection. Rodents are the most plausible candidates for the monkeypox natural reservoir, however, this has not yet been determined. Eating undercooked meat and other diseased animal products is a potential risk factor. People who live in or close to forests may be indirectly or minimally exposed to diseased animals.

Close contact with respiratory secretions, skin sores on an infected person, or recently contaminated items may cause human-to-human transmission. Health professionals, family members, and other close contacts of current patients are more at risk because droplet respiratory particles often need extended face-to-face contact.

The number of person-to-person infections in a community's longest recorded chain of transmission has increased from 6 to 9 in recent years. This could be an indication of a general decline in immunity brought on by the end of smallpox vaccination campaigns. Congenital monkeypox may result through transmission via the placenta, which can also happen during intimate contact during labor and after delivery. Although close physical contact is a recognized risk factor for transmission, it is not known at this time whether monkeypox may particularly spread via sexual intercourse. Studies are required to comprehend this danger better.

Chapter 5: key facts and Question on Monkeypox

Key facts:

The monkeypox vaccines employed in the smallpox eradication operation also offered protection against that disease. One of the more recent vaccinations that have been created is licensed to prevent monkeypox.

The monkeypox virus, a species of the Orthopoxvirus genus in the family Poxviridae, is the culprit behind monkeypox.

Typically, monkeypox is a self-limiting illness with symptoms that last between two and four weeks. There may be severe instances. The case fatality rate has recently been in the range of 3-6%.

Humans may get monkeypox through coming into intimate contact with an animal or person who has the disease, as well as by coming into touch with contaminated objects.

By coming into intimate contact with lesions, bodily fluids, respiratory droplets, and infected objects like bedding, the monkeypox virus may spread from one person to another.

A viral zoonotic illness called monkeypox is most common in tropical rainforest regions of central and west Africa, with sporadic exportations to other places.

Monkeypox has been officially treated using an antiviral drug that was originally used to treat smallpox.

Monkeypox has a clinical appearance similar to smallpox, an orthopoxvirus infection that was eliminated globally in 1980. Compared to smallpox, monkeypox is less infectious and has milder symptoms.

Clinical symptoms of monkeypox often include fever, rash, and enlarged lymph nodes, and it may result in a variety of health issues.

Frequently Asked Questions On Monkeypox

Describe monkeypox.

The monkeypox virus is the infection that causes monkeypox. It may transmit from animals to people since it is a viral zoonotic illness. It may also pass from one individual to another.

What signs and symptoms manifest in monkeypox?

Numerous symptoms and indicators are associated with monkeypox. While some individuals only have minor symptoms, others may experience more severe symptoms and need medical attention. Pregnant women, children, and anyone with impaired immune systems are at increased risk for serious illness or complications.

Monkeypox is most often characterized by fever, headache, muscular pains, back discomfort, lack of energy, and enlarged lymph nodes. A rash that may continue for two to three weeks develops as a result of or in conjunction with this. The face, palms of the hands, soles of the feet, eyes, mouth, throat, groin, and genital and/or anal parts of the body may all be affected by the rash. Lesions may number anywhere from one to thousands. Lesions start flat, fill with fluids, then crust over, dry up, and fall off, revealing a new layer of skin underneath.

Symptoms normally last two to three weeks and disappear on their own or with supportive treatment, such as fever-relieving drugs or painkillers. Until all lesions have crusted over, all scabs have fallen off, and a fresh layer of skin has developed below, a person is still contagious. Anyone who may have monkeypox symptoms or who has come into touch with someone who has should contact or see a healthcare professional for guidance.

Can monkeypox cause fatal illness or severe illness in humans?

Monkeypox symptoms often disappear on their own in a few weeks. An infection, however, may sometimes result in serious health issues or even death. Monkeypox may cause more severe symptoms and even death in newborns, toddlers, and persons with underlying immune weaknesses.

Monkeypox may lead to more skin infections, pneumonia, disorientation, and vision issues. In the past, between 1% and 10% of monkeypox victims have perished. It is important to remember that mortality rates in various contexts may vary as a result of a variety of circumstances, including access to healthcare. Due to historically low levels of monitoring for monkeypox, these numbers might be inflated. There have been no fatalities yet in the recently afflicted nations where the current epidemic is occurring.

How is monkeypox transmitted from one person to another?

Close contact with someone who has a monkeypox rash, such as by face-to-face, skin-to-skin, mouth-to-mouth, or mouth-to-skin contact, including sexual contact, may transfer the disease from one person to another. Monkeypox sufferers are typically infectious until all of their lesions have crusted over, the scabs have gone off, and a new layer of skin has developed below. However, we are still discovering how long monkeypox sufferers remain contagious.

Monkeypox virus contamination may occur in environments, such as when an infected individual touches items including clothes, bedding, towels, gadgets, and surfaces. If someone else comes in contact with these things, they might become sick. It's also possible to get a virus via clothes, bedding, or towels, or by breathing in skin flakes. Transmission of the fomite is what this is.

The virus may spread by direct contact with the mouth, respiratory droplets, and perhaps through short-range aerosols if there are ulcers, lesions, or sores in the mouth. Monkeypox transmission via the air may occur for unknown reasons, and research is being done to find out more.

The virus may also pass from a pregnant person to the fetus, from a newborn to a parent via intimate contact, or from a parent who has monkeypox to a kid.

Although cases of asymptomatic illness have been documented, it is unclear whether or not contagious diseases may be disseminated by asymptomatic individuals or by other body fluids. Semen has been confirmed to contain monkeypox viral DNA, however, it is unknown whether semen, vaginal fluids, amniotic fluids, lactation, or blood may also transmit the illness. The question of whether persons may transmit monkeypox via the sharing of these fluids during and after symptomatic illness is now being researched.

Is monkeypox transmitted from animals to people?

When a person comes into touch with an infected animal, they risk contracting monkeypox. Primates and rodents are examples of animal hosts. By staying away from unprotected contact with wild animals, particularly those that are ill or dead, the chance of contracting monkeypox from them may be decreased (including their meat and blood). All items containing animal flesh or parts should be fully prepared before consumption in monkeypox-endemic nations.

Is it possible for people to transmit monkeypox to animals?

Although no cases of humans spreading monkeypox to animals have been recorded, it is a possibility. Avoid close contact with all animals, including pets (such as cats, dogs, hamsters, gerbils, etc.), livestock, and wildlife, if you have proven or suspect monkeypox. Animals known to be vulnerable to the monkeypox virus, such as rats and non-human primates, should be avoided by people with monkeypox.

Who is susceptible to monkeypox?

The most vulnerable groups of people are those who often interact with potentially infected animals or those who live with or have intimate contact (including sexual contact) with a person who has a monkeypox. While caring for patients with monkeypox, health professionals should adhere to infection prevention and control procedures to keep themselves safe.

In rare instances, monkeypox may cause mortality in newborns, young children, and those with underlying immune weaknesses. These individuals may have more severe symptoms.

Those who had the smallpox vaccine may be somewhat protected against monkeypox.

However, it is improbable that younger individuals received the smallpox vaccine since, when the disease was declared eliminated in most of the globe in 1980, immunization programs were discontinued. Those who have received the smallpox vaccine should continue to take preventative measures to safeguard both themselves and others.

How can I prevent monkeypox from spreading to other people?

By avoiding direct contact with people or animals that may be afflicted with the disease, you may lessen your chance of contracting monkeypox. Frequently clean and disinfect any areas that may have been infected with a virus from an infectious person. Keep yourself aware of the prevalence of monkeypox in your community and be upfront with anyone you come into close contact with (particularly during sexual activity) about any symptoms you or they may be experiencing.

By obtaining medical assistance and keeping to yourself until you have been examined and tested, you may take precautions to protect others if you believe you may have monkeypox. You should keep to yourself if you have monkeypox until all of your lesions have crusted over, the scabs have come off, and a new layer of skin has developed below if you have monkeypox that has been diagnosed as probable or proven. You won't be able to spread the infection to others as a result of this. Ask your health professional for guidance on whether you should isolate yourself at home or a medical institution. Use condoms as a precaution while having sexual contact for 12 weeks after you have recovered until more is known regarding the transfer of sexually transmitted diseases via sexual fluids.

What should I do if I suspect I have monkeypox symptoms or have come into contact with someone who does?

If you have been in close contact with someone who has monkeypox or has been in a location where the virus may have been present, keep a watchful eye out for symptoms for 21 days following your last exposure. As much as possible, avoid having close personal interactions with others, but if it's necessary, let them know that you've just been exposed to monkeypox.

For guidance, evaluation, and medical attention, speak with your healthcare professional if you believe you may be experiencing monkeypox symptoms. If you can, keep yourself alone until you get the results of your exam. Keep your hands clean.

If you test positive for monkeypox, your doctor will give you advice on how to treat the infection, whether you should isolate yourself at home or in a hospital.

I have monkeypox; what should I do to prevent spreading the disease to others?

Your doctor will recommend whether you should get treatment in a hospital or at home if you have monkeypox. This will depend on the severity of your symptoms, whether you have risk factors that put you at risk for more severe symptoms, and if you can reduce the chance that everyone you live with will get infected.

If staying home alone is suggested, you shouldn't leave the house. Protect those you share a home with as much as you can by:

Being secluded in a different room

use a separate restroom, or after each use, clean it

Avoid sweeping or vacuuming and instead clean regularly touched surfaces with soap, water, and a home disinfectant (this might disturb virus particles and cause others to become infected) use distinct dishes, towels, beds, and gadgets.

Doing your laundry (carefully lifting bedding, clothing, and towels without shaking them, placing items in plastic bags before transporting them to the washer, and washing them in hot water of more than 60 degrees).

window openings for effective ventilation.

encourage everyone in the household to routinely wash their hands with soap and water or hand sanitizer that contains alcohol.

Do your best to reduce their danger if you can't avoid being in the same room as someone else or being close to someone else when you're alone at home by:

avoiding physical contact

Frequently wash your hands

wearing garments or applying bandages on your rash.

Make sure you and anybody in the room with you are wearing properly fitted medical masks and opening windows around the house.

keeping a minimum distance of 1 meter.

If you are unable to wash your laundry and someone else has to do it for you, you should wear a medical mask that fits comfortably, disposable gloves, and follow the aforementioned laundry safety procedures.

Is the monkeypox vaccination available?

Yes. Recently, a vaccination for monkeypox was licensed. For those who are at risk, several nations advise immunization. For the smallpox illness, which has been eliminated, better and safer vaccinations have been developed. These vaccines may also be helpful for monkeypox. One of these has been authorized for use in monkeypox prophylaxis. Only those who are vulnerable should be thought about being vaccinated, such as those who have had intimate contact with someone who has monkeypox. At this time, mass immunization is not advised.

Although smallpox vaccination has been protective against monkeypox in the past, there is currently minimal information on the efficacy of more recent smallpox/monkeypox vaccines in preventing monkeypox in clinical settings and the field. It will be possible to quickly generate new data on the efficacy of these vaccinations in various contexts by examining the usage of monkeypox vaccines wherever they are used.

How is the monkeypox disease treated?

People who have monkeypox should heed their doctor's instructions. Treatment is often not necessary since symptoms usually go away on their own. Analgesics and antipyretics, which are used to treat fever and discomfort, may be used to ease certain symptoms. Anyone suffering from monkeypox should drink enough fluids, eat healthfully, and get plenty of rest.

Self-isolating individuals should take care of their mental health by engaging in activities that they find enjoyable and relaxing, staying in touch with loved ones via technology, engaging in physical activity if they feel well enough to do so while isolating, and seeking support for their mental health if necessary.

Monkeypox patients should refrain from scratching their rash and take care of it by washing their hands before and after handling the lesions and by keeping their skin dry and uncovered (unless they are unavoidably in a room with someone else, in which case they should cover it with clothing or a bandage until they can isolate again). Sterilized water or an antiseptic solution may be used to keep the rash clean. Mouth lesions may be treated with salt water rinses, while body lesions can be treated with warm Epsom salt and baking soda baths. Pain relief from oral and perianal lesions is possible with lidocaine application.

Products that may help treat monkeypox have been developed as a result of years of study on smallpox therapies. The European Medicines Agency authorized tecovirimat, an antiviral originally developed to treat smallpox, in January 2022 to treat monkeypox. There is limited experience using these therapeutics during a monkeypox outbreak. Because of this, gathering information to help with future use is often done in conjunction with their use.

Where is monkeypox now a concern in the world?

Monkeypox is presently spreading throughout many nations in regions where the virus has not previously been detected, including Europe, the Americas, Africa, the Western Pacific, and nations in the Eastern Mediterranean. In areas of Africa that have previously recorded occurrences, such as Nigeria, the Democratic Republic of the Congo, and the Central African Republic, more cases than usual have been reported in 2022. WHO is collaborating with all impacted nations to improve monitoring, provide advice on how to limit the spread, and provide medical treatment.

Before this epidemic, reports of monkeypox were made in a few African nations. These include Gabon, Cameroon, Liberia, Nigeria, Sierra Leone, the Democratic Republic of the Congo, the Central African Republic, the Republic of the Congo, Côte d'Ivoire, and the Central African

Republic. Some of these nations only had a small number of cases, whereas others saw ongoing or repeated outbreaks. Travel from Nigeria has been connected to rare incidents in other nations. The current epidemic, which is impacting several nations at once, is unlike earlier outbreaks.

Cases of monkeypox have been recorded in several nations that generally do not have them in 2022, why?

The majority of infections in this outbreak—but not all—are among males who engage in sexual activity with other men who have recently had intercourse with a new partner or partners. Fewer symptoms are often recorded than what was customarily seen in the past. Please visit this page for the most recent information on the number of cases and the nations that are reporting cases.

As of July 11, 2022, no connection has been made between the majority of cases that have been reported on an individual basis with travel from previously afflicted nations in Africa. In this epidemic, recent travel from different parts of the globe is often mentioned.

We recognize that many people are worried about this epidemic, particularly those whose loved ones or communities have been impacted. The most important thing at this time is to educate those who are most susceptible to monkeypox and provide tips on how to stop future transmission between individuals. Additionally, public health professionals must be able to recognize, classify, and treat patients.

Because anybody may get monkeypox and stigmatization can weaken control efforts, no one must stigmatize anyone who is impacted by this outbreak. In impacted nations, WHO is striving to provide the Member States with instruments for monkeypox monitoring, preparation, and outbreak response.

To better understand how individuals are exposed to monkeypox, studies are being conducted in the afflicted nations. Medical attention is being given to people who are harmed, and public health initiatives are being established to stop the spread of the disease.

Is there a chance that this epidemic might go farther?

Because it must be passed from person to person, skin to skin, mouth to skin, or mouth to mouth to spread, a contaminated environment, or an infected animal, monkeypox is less infectious than certain other illnesses. We have a window of opportunity to stem the spread of this epidemic by collaborating closely with communities and groups that are more vulnerable. Everyone must cooperate right away to halt the spread by being aware of their risk and taking steps to reduce it.

To stop the pandemic from spreading further, WHO is taking immediate action. The WHO's top priorities include finding out more about the virus's mode of transmission during this epidemic and preventing other individuals from contracting the disease. Stopping the spread of this new problem will be made easier by increasing awareness of it.

What do we know about sex and monkeypox?

Monkeypox may be shared by any form of intimate contact, including kissing, touching, oral, penetrative vaginal, or anal intercourse with an infected person. Before being tested for monkeypox and STIs, anybody with new or unusual skin lesions or rashes should refrain from initiating sexual activity.

Chickenpox, herpes, and syphilis are just a few infectious diseases that monkeypox might mimic. This may help to explain why several infections in the ongoing epidemic have been linked to patients at sexual health clinics. Do not forget that the rash may also appear in areas that are difficult to views, such as the mouth, throat, genitalia, vagina, and anus/anal region.

Although the monkeypox virus has been discovered in semen, it is still unknown whether or not semen or vaginal secretions may transmit the disease. After recovering from monkeypox, patients are encouraged to wear condoms for 12 weeks until more is known about the virus's prevalence and potential for infectivity in semen. Monkeypox cannot be prevented, but using a condom may help protect you and others from a variety of other STIs.

If at all feasible, provide your new sexual partners—even those you didn't want to see again—with your contact information. This will enable you to be informed if your spouse exhibits any symptoms or to alert them if it affects you. Multiple sexual partners are urged to take precautions to lower their chance of exposure by avoiding close contact with someone exhibiting symptoms. Your risk will be lower if you have fewer sexual partners.

Any sort of intimate contact with an affected person may transmit the virus, not only via sexual interaction. Residents in the same home are more vulnerable. Anyone who suspects they may have monkeypox should see a health professional very once.

Who has the increased chance of contracting monkeypox?

Sexually active people or guys who have sex with males are not the only ones who run the danger of getting monkeypox. Those who are close to someone who exhibits symptoms are in danger.

In this epidemic, many of the cases that have been reported have been found in males who have intercourse with other guys. Males who have sex with men may now be at increased risk of exposure if they have close contact with an infected individual given that the virus is currently spreading from person to person in these social networks.

At sexual health clinics, monkeypox cases have been discovered sometimes. One explanation for the present increase in reports of monkeypox cases among communities of men who have sex with men might be attributed to this population's proactive pursuit of health. Herpes and syphilis are two sexually transmitted illnesses that monkeypox rashes might mimic, which may help to explain why these instances are being discovered at sexual health clinics. As we get more knowledge, we could find additional examples in the larger community.

To protect individuals who are most in danger, it is crucial to include communities of homosexual, bisexual, and other men who have sex with males in awareness campaigns. Know your risk if you have intercourse with other males as a man, and take precautions to safeguard both yourself and others. Anyone who thinks they may have monkeypox should see a doctor right once to be tested and get therapy.

If I have HIV, is there a larger chance that I may get monkeypox, show severe symptoms, or die away?

Close interaction with a person who has monkeypox puts others at risk of contracting the disease. HIV may compromise your immune system if it is not treated. There is some evidence to suggest that having a damaged immune system may raise your chance of contracting the disease if exposed, developing a severe illness, or passing away from monkeypox. To properly appreciate this, however, further information is required.

Those who have underlying immune weaknesses may be more susceptible to monkeypox-related disease. People with HIV may achieve viral suppression if they are aware of their status, have access to therapy, and utilize it as directed. This indicates that, compared to when individuals were not receiving therapy, their immune systems are less susceptible to additional illnesses. There have been many HIV-positive individuals in the current epidemic, but there have been few serious cases, perhaps because their HIV infection was under control. Studies are being conducted to learn more about these issues.

People with many sexual partners, including those with HIV, are urged to take precautions to lessen their chance of contracting monkeypox by keeping a safe distance from anybody exhibiting symptoms. Having fewer sexual partners might lower your risk.

Is having COVID-19 or long-COVID a risk factor for developing monkeypox or experiencing severe symptoms from it?

Health experts are actively working to find a solution to this query. Whether having COVID-19 or a post-COVID-19 condition (long-COVID) renders you more susceptible to monkeypox is unknown at this time. More research is required on individuals who now have monkeypox or who have COVID-19 infection or a post-COVID-19 condition.

If you already have COVID-19, abide by WHO recommendations. Avoid contact with others to stop the virus from spreading, and keep an eye on your symptoms so you can obtain the proper treatment. Contact a health professional if you believe you have a post-COVID problem to obtain the assistance you need.

What can I do to lessen the load on my local sex workers, who are overworked?

By taking steps to maintain your health, such as engaging in safer sex, you may help your community's health services. Utilizing online, video or phone services that are suitable and accessible for your queries or symptoms helps ease the burden on in-person services. By taking precautions against monkeypox, you may lessen the number of cases, put a stop to the epidemic, and lessen the strain on healthcare systems.

Even if they are busy, you must get in touch with a healthcare professional for guidance, testing, and treatment if you have symptoms that might be monkeypox. Because monkeypox spreads via close contact, take precautions to prevent infecting medical staff. Wear a mask, cover your skin with clothes, and phone ahead before your appointment to let them know you think your symptoms could be related to monkeypox.

Can kids acquire monkeypox?

If a child comes into intimate touch with a person who is exhibiting symptoms, they may get monkeypox. Children are often more susceptible to serious illness than adolescents and adults, according to data from previously impacted nations. In the most recent epidemic, a small number of kids have had monkeypox.

What should I do if a kid in my care exhibits signs of monkeypox?

The rash associated with monkeypox might mirror that of other viral diseases and other common pediatric illnesses like chickenpox. Consult a healthcare professional if a kid in your care exhibits symptoms that might indicate monkeypox. They will assist in getting them checked and the treatment they need.

Serious monkeypox may be more common in children than in adults. Until they are well, they should be continuously watched in case they need more care. The child's health worker may suggest that they get treated in a medical institution. In this case, they will be permitted to isolate themselves with a parent or caregiver who is healthy and at low risk of monkeypox.

Which hazards are associated with monkeypox during pregnancy?

The hazards of monkeypox during pregnancy and how the virus may be transmitted to the fetus in the womb, the newborn during or after delivery, or a nursing infant require more study. According to the knowledge that is currently available, getting monkeypox while pregnant may be harmful to the baby.

Avoid close contact with somebody who has monkeypox if you are pregnant. No matter who they are, everyone who comes into touch with an infected person may acquire monkeypox.

Contact your healthcare practitioner if you believe you may have been exposed to monkeypox or if you exhibit symptoms that may be monkeypox. They will assist in getting you tested and the treatment you need.

If I have been diagnosed with monkeypox, can I still breastfeed?

Ask your healthcare practitioner for guidance if you have monkeypox that has been confirmed or if you believe you may have. Both the danger of spreading monkeypox and the risk of not nursing your child will be evaluated. They will give you advice on how to lower the risk by taking precautions including covering your lesions and wearing a mask to limit the danger of passing on the virus if you can continue breastfeeding and maintain close contact.

It will be important to carefully weigh the danger of infection against the possible damage and suffering brought on by stopping nursing and maintaining close contact between parent and child. There has to be more research done to determine if the monkeypox virus may pass from mom to kid via breastfeeding.

Why is this illness referred to as "monkeypox"?

Because it was initially discovered in 1958 in colonies of monkeys held for study, the illness is sometimes known as monkeypox. Only later, in 1970, was it discovered in humans.

Is it possible for the monkeypox virus to spread by blood transfusion?

Never donate blood if you're feeling under the weather. If you are scheduled to donate blood, evaluate your health beforehand, keep an eye out for monkeypox symptoms, and postpone your appointment if necessary.

When individuals may donate blood, there are severe rules in place. The potential donor is questioned about their present state of health and any symptoms they may be having. This lowers the possibility of someone with an infectious condition donating blood.

Does prior chickenpox exposure provide any defense against monkeypox?

A separate virus causes chickenpox (the varicella virus). Past chickenpox exposure does not provide protection against monkeypox (caused by the monkeypox virus, which is an orthodox virus).

Is there a test to determine whether I've ever had monkeypox?

Some tests can determine if you have orthopoxvirus antibodies (the family of viruses that monkeypox belongs to). These tests may assist in determining if you have ever had an orthopoxvirus exposure or had smallpox or monkeypox vaccination. The tests, however, are unable to determine if you were previously exposed to the monkeypox virus, a vaccination, or another orthopoxvirus. Because of this, antibody testing is not often used to diagnose suspected new cases of monkeypox or screen for prior exposure to the disease.

I've previously had monkeypox. Can I catch it once more?

Currently, nothing is known about the duration of immunity after monkeypox infection. The extent to which having had monkeypox in the past confers protection against subsequent infections and for how long if at all, is still unclear. Even if you've already had monkeypox, you should take every precaution to prevent re-infection.

You can safeguard others by taking on the role of designated caregiver if you have had monkeypox in the past and someone in your home has it now. This is because you are more likely than others to have some immunity. To prevent contracting an infection, you should still take all necessary measures.

Why was monkeypox deemed a worldwide public health emergency?

On July 23, 2022, Dr. Tedros Adhanom Ghebreyesus, Director-General of WHO, proclaimed the multi-nation monkeypox epidemic to be a public health emergency of global concern (PHEIC). The International Health Regulations' highest degree of public health alert, the declaration of a PHEIC, may strengthen coordination, collaboration, and international solidarity.

A well-planned reaction may halt the spread of disease and save vulnerable populations.

Additionally, the Director-General issued Temporary Recommendations to assist nations in containing and battling the spread. You may read the Director-complete General's statement and see his list of recommendations here.

Since the outbreak started to spread in early May 2022, WHO has taken this extraordinary situation very seriously. As a result, it has issued public health and clinical guidance quickly, actively engaged with communities, and gathered hundreds of scientists and researchers to advance research on monkeypox and the potential for the creation of new diagnostics, vaccines, and treatments.